Emergency contact:

Insurance Information

Insurance Information

Doctor List

Pharmacy List

Health Care Directive Information

Lawyers

Current/Previous Conditions

Special Instructions:

Allergy List

Previous Hospital Stays/ Surgeries

Medication Name	Dose	Frequency

New Symptoms

Improvements

Drs Appointments

Referrals Needed

Medicine Refills

Information to Research/ Things to do

Medical Questions

Notes:

Follow up:

New Symptoms

Improvements

Drs Appointments

Referrals Needed

Medicine Refills

Information to Research/ Things to do

Medical Questions

Notes:

Follow up:

New Symptoms

Improvements

Drs Appointments

Referrals Needed

Medicine Refills

Information to Research/ Things to do

Medical Questions

Notes:

Follow up:

New Symptoms

Improvements

Drs Appointments

Referrals Needed

Medicine Refills

Information to Research/ Things to do

Medical Questions

Notes:

Follow up:

New Symptoms

Improvements

Drs Appointments

Referrals Needed

Medicine Refills

Information to Research/ Things to do

Medical Questions

Notes:

Follow up:

New Symptoms

Improvements

Drs Appointments

Referrals Needed

Medicine Refills

Information to Research/ Things to do

Medical Questions

Notes:

Follow up:

New Symptoms

Improvements

Drs Appointments

Referrals Needed

Medicine Refills

Information to Research/ Things to do

Medical Questions

Notes:

Follow up:

New Symptoms

Improvements

Drs Appointments   Referrals Needed   Medicine Refills

Information to Research/ Things to do

Medical Questions

Notes:

Follow up:

New Symptoms

Improvements

Drs Appointments

Referrals Needed

Medicine Refills

Information to Research/ Things to do

Medical Questions

Notes:

Follow up:

New Symptoms

Improvements

Drs Appointments   Referrals Needed   Medicine Refills

Information to Research/ Things to do

Medical Questions

Notes:

Follow up:

New Symptoms

Improvements

Drs Appointments	Referrals Needed	Medicine Refills

Information to Research/ Things to do

Medical Questions

Notes:

Follow up:

New Symptoms

Improvements

Drs Appointments

Referrals Needed

Medicine Refills

Information to Research/ Things to do

Medical Questions

Notes:

Follow up:

New Symptoms

Improvements

Drs Appointments   Referrals Needed   Medicine Refills

Information to Research/ Things to do

Medical Questions

Notes:

Follow up:

New Symptoms

Improvements

Drs Appointments

Referrals Needed

Medicine Refills

Information to Research/ Things to do

Medical Questions

Notes:

Follow up:

New Symptoms

Improvements

Drs Appointments   Referrals Needed   Medicine Refills

Information to Research/ Things to do

Medical Questions

Notes:

Follow up:

New Symptoms

Improvements

Drs Appointments

Referrals Needed

Medicine Refills

Information to Research/ Things to do

Medical Questions

Notes:

Follow up:

New Symptoms

Improvements

Drs Appointments   Referrals Needed   Medicine Refills

Information to Research/ Things to do

Medical Questions

Notes:

Follow up:

New Symptoms

Improvements

Drs Appointments

Referrals Needed

Medicine Refills

Information to Research/ Things to do

Medical Questions

Notes:

Follow up:

New Symptoms

Improvements

Drs Appointments   Referrals Needed   Medicine Refills

Information to Research/ Things to do

Medical Questions

Notes:

Follow up:

New Symptoms

Improvements

Drs Appointments   Referrals Needed   Medicine Refills

Information to Research/ Things to do

Medical Questions

Notes:

Follow up:

New Symptoms

Improvements

Drs Appointments

Referrals Needed

Medicine Refills

Information to Research/ Things to do

Medical Questions

Notes:

Follow up:

New Symptoms

Improvements

Drs Appointments   Referrals Needed   Medicine Refills

Information to Research/ Things to do

Medical Questions

Notes:

Follow up:

New Symptoms

Improvements

Drs Appointments   Referrals Needed   Medicine Refills

Information to Research/ Things to do

Medical Questions

Notes:

Follow up:

New Symptoms

Improvements

Drs Appointments

Referrals Needed

Medicine Refills

Information to Research/ Things to do

Medical Questions

Notes:

Follow up:

New Symptoms

Improvements

Drs Appointments

Referrals Needed

Medicine Refills

Information to Research/ Things to do

Medical Questions

Notes:

Follow up:

New Symptoms

Improvements

Drs Appointments	Referrals Needed	Medicine Refills

Information to Research/ Things to do

Medical Questions

Notes:

Follow up:

New Symptoms

Improvements

Drs Appointments

Referrals Needed

Medicine Refills

Information to Research/ Things to do

Medical Questions

Notes:

Follow up:

New Symptoms

Improvements

Drs Appointments	Referrals Needed	Medicine Refills

Information to Research/ Things to do

Medical Questions

Notes:

Follow up:

New Symptoms

Improvements

Drs Appointments

Referrals Needed

Medicine Refills

Information to Research/ Things to do

Medical Questions

Notes:

Follow up:

New Symptoms

Improvements

Drs Appointments

Referrals Needed

Medicine Refills

Information to Research/ Things to do

Medical Questions

Notes:

Follow up:

New Symptoms

Improvements

Drs Appointments

Referrals Needed

Medicine Refills

Information to Research/ Things to do

Medical Questions

Notes:

Follow up:

New Symptoms

Improvements

Drs Appointments

Referrals Needed

Medicine Refills

Information to Research/ Things to do

Medical Questions

Notes:

Follow up:

New Symptoms

Improvements

Drs Appointments   Referrals Needed   Medicine Refills

Information to Research/ Things to do

Medical Questions

Notes:

Follow up:

New Symptoms

Improvements

Drs Appointments   ## Referrals Needed   ## Medicine Refills

Information to Research/ Things to do

Medical Questions

Notes:

Follow up:

New Symptoms

Improvements

Drs Appointments	Referrals Needed	Medicine Refills

Information to Research/ Things to do

Medical Questions

Notes:

Follow up:

New Symptoms

Improvements

Drs Appointments

Referrals Needed

Medicine Refills

Information to Research/ Things to do

Medical Questions

Notes:

Follow up:

Hospitalizations

Medical Questions

Notes:

Follow up:

Notes

Medical Questions

Notes:

Follow up:

Notes

Medical Questions

Notes:

Follow up:

Notes

Medical Questions

Notes:

Follow up:

Notes

Medical Questions

Notes:

Follow up:

Notes

Medical Questions

Notes:

Follow up:

Notes

Notes

Medical Questions

Notes:

Follow up:

Notes

Medical Questions

Notes:

Follow up:

Notes

Medical Questions

Notes:

Follow up:

Notes

Medical Questions

Notes:

Follow up:

Notes

Medical Questions

Notes:

Follow up:

Notes

Medical Questions

Notes:

Follow up:

Notes

Medical Questions

Notes:

Follow up:

Notes

Medical Questions

Notes:

Follow up:

Notes

Medical Questions

Notes:

Follow up:

Notes

Medical Questions

Notes:

Follow up:

Notes

Medical Questions

Notes:

Follow up:

Notes

Notes

Medical Questions

Notes:

Follow up:

Notes

Medical Questions

Notes:

Follow up:

Notes

Medical Questions

Notes:

Follow up:

Notes

Medical Questions

Notes:

Follow up:

Notes

Medical Questions

Notes:

Follow up:

Notes

Medical Questions

Notes:

Follow up:

Notes

Medical Questions

Notes:

Follow up:

Notes

Medical Questions

Notes:

Follow up:

Notes

Medical Questions

Notes:

Follow up:

Notes

Medical Questions

Notes:

Follow up:

Notes

Medical Questions

Notes:

Follow up:

Notes

Medical Questions

Notes:

Follow up:

Notes

Medical Questions

Notes:

Follow up:

Notes

Medical Questions

Notes:

Follow up:

Notes

Medical Questions

Notes:

Follow up:

Notes

Medical Questions

Notes:

Follow up:

Notes

Medical Questions

Notes:

Follow up:

Notes

Medical Questions

Notes:

Follow up:

Notes

Medical Questions

Notes:

Follow up:

Notes

Medical Questions

Notes:

Follow up:

Notes

Medical Questions

Notes:

Follow up:

Notes

Medical Questions

Notes:

Follow up:

Notes

Medical Questions

Notes:

Follow up:

Notes

Medical Questions

Notes:

Follow up:

Notes

Medical Questions

Notes:

Follow up:

Notes

Medical Questions

Notes:

Follow up:

Notes

Medical Questions

Notes:

Follow up:

Notes

Medical Questions

Notes:

Follow up:

Notes